Cognitive Behavioral Therapy

Worksheets for Substance Abuse

Self and Group CBT Activities Workbook to Manage Drugs Addiction, Prevent Relapse and Treatment Planner

Portia Cruise

Disclaimer

Personal Details

Name:	
Age:	
Diagnosed Issue	
Phone Number:	
Emergency Contact Number:	
Mental Health Institute	
Dr. in Charge	

Introduction

Congratulations on getting this workbook that uses the CBT model to deal with the substance abuse challenge. You got this workbook because you or someone you love wants to kick out their drug addiction problem.

This workbook uses the **PLAN-DO-ACT-FEEDBACK** model to help you fight this habit in an organized way. By using the metrics in this book, you will be able to track your success as you work your way on the journey ahead of you. Like in many endeavors in life including fighting substance abuse addiction, without a way to measure your progress, you can never know how far you have come or gone. Because progress usually seems slow at first, many people give up just when they should really be intensifying their efforts.

This worksheet will help you monitor the progress of your therapy using Cognitive Behavioral Therapy in this logbook, it is a self-help book that can help you manage your thoughts better so that you are better able to control your emotions and your behavior. It is an essential tool for cognitive therapy that contains a series of questions aimed at guiding you step-by-step through the process of identifying your negative thinking and changing them.

Experience has shown that it is better to enter the details of your activity into the logbook as soon as is possible when the information is still fresh in your memory.

This logbook is more than just a record of your thought records, it also covers your action plans and possible improvement you plan to undertake.

This substance abuse self-help Worksheets Therapy book is a reliable partner in your journey to get the best out of your Therapeutic sessions.

Good Luck in your healing process!!!

About This Workbook

This workbook is divided into three parts

1. Personal Insight

Uncovering your Insight is the key point in dealing with addiction. This portion consists of several activities and questions that make you more clear about the sensitivity and the severity of the problem. It will give you a deeper understanding of the problem and motivates you to continue the process of achieving a drug-free life. Try to complete each sheet with truth and full peace of mind

2. Overcoming Addiction

This is the practical portion of the workbook. It includes different activities that help you to set realistic and achievable goals, find out red and safe zone and challenge unhealthy thoughts, feelings, and emotions. This section aims to help you understand why he/she feels or acts in certain ways and how these feelings and actions lead to substance abuse. This portion will equip you with the right tools to overcome addiction

3. Maintaining a Healthy Life

This is one of the most tricky parts of the whole process to be drug-free after completing the treatment. Management and relapse prevention go side by side as the person is prone to relapse at any stage of recovery. This will help you to develop strategies and coping mechanisms to deal with the Red Alerts of relapse. In the end, the person develops the confidence to handle the challenging situation without abusing substance

Using this Workbook

This self-help workbook contains worksheets to help you in your fight against substance abuse. Individual and peer therapy groups. It is written in a very simple language that anyone can understand.

You start by filling the self-assessment section and then measure how much substance abuse affects you.

Following the section for accessing motivation is the section where you get to write out both the long and short-term Costs and Benefits of stopping your substance abuse problem.

Then you have to color the pie chart to estimate how your substance abuse affects the different aspects of your life.

Next, you get to record how strong your cravings for substance are. Each of these has to be recorded daily.

With the personal profiling over, the worksheet will now begin at this point. To make you get the most out of this workbook, it has been divided into Week 1, Week 2, Week 3, and Week 4.

In each of those weeks, you will have to identify those things that increase your chances of relapsing despite all your efforts.

You will also be introduced to the Addiction Model popularly used in CBT therapy. The Addiction Model is used in with the thought changing process to challenge the first thought that you had when you were triggered by your experience that made you crave drugs.

You can find more details in the appendix.

Overcoming Substance Abuse

A Self-help Workbook

Workbook Includes:

■ Self-Assessment

■ Insight of Problem

■ Motivation Check

■ Cost Benefit Analysis

■ Goals of Treatment

■ Craving Record

■ Relapse Prevention

■ Dealing with Risk

■ Thought and Behavior

■ Challenge Negative Thoughts

■ Addiction Model

■ Emotion Management

■ Review

Self Assessment

Answer **yes** or **no**

1. Do you feel guilty after abusing substance? ☐

2. Are your sleep and appetite effected because of substance abuse? ☐

3. Do you neglect your job/ business because of substance abuse? ☐

4. Does substance abuse affect your relationship and family life? ☐

5. Do you sometimes feel people avoid you because of substance abuse? ☐

6. Has your reputation been negatively affected by substance abuse? ☐

7. Have you ever felt the need to reduce your substance intake? ☐

8. Does your work efficacy reduce from substance abuse? ☐

9. Does your craving for substance abuse forced you to an instant dose? ☐

10. Do you feel sharper senses after abusing substance? ☐

11. Have you ever felt that your regular intake doesn't satisfy so you increase your quantity? ☐

12. Do you think substance abuse makes you care less about your family and relationship? ☐

13. Have you ever been in hospital because of substance abuse? ☐

Instructions

This is a very important first step in this journey. In this step, you do a self-examination. The answers to the questions above will serve as a guide. You can also generate your own questions

Severity of Problems

How serious do you consider this substance abuse problem? Is it low, moderate, high, severe, or extreme?

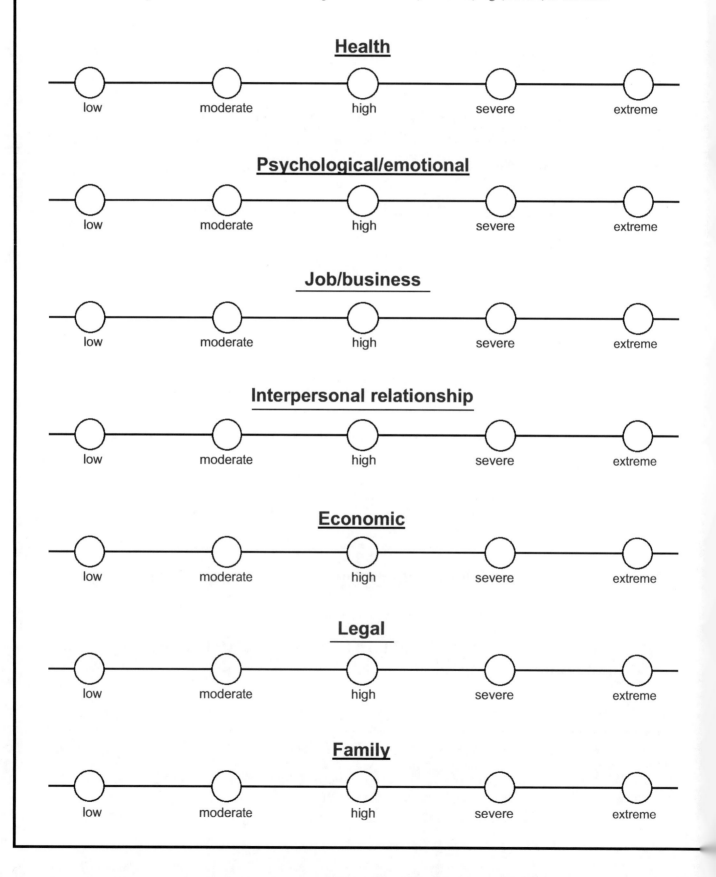

Health

low   moderate   high   severe   extreme

Psychological/emotional

low   moderate   high   severe   extreme

Job/business

low   moderate   high   severe   extreme

Interpersonal relationship

low   moderate   high   severe   extreme

Economic

low   moderate   high   severe   extreme

Legal

low   moderate   high   severe   extreme

Family

low   moderate   high   severe   extreme

Motivation Check

I'm ready to quit (if the answer is 'no' skip this section) because...

Describe in detail the most important reason to quit

Describe in detail the challenges you may face

Motivation Check

I'm not ready to quit (skip this section if you have already answered the previous section) because...

Describe in detail the biggest hurdle

Cost Benefit Analysis

Immediate Result

Cost of Using

What do you consider the most instant consequences of your drug abuse?

Benefits of Using

What do you consider the most instant benefits of your drug usage?

Long Term Result

Cost of Using

What do you consider the most long-term consequences of your drug abuse, many months, or years from now?

Benefits of Using

What do you consider the most long-term benefits of your drug abuse, many months, or years from now?

Goals of Treatment

Set measurable goals with a time frame

Physical	Goals	Strategies

Physical goals can include a reduction of your drug intake by a specific amount and at a specific time

■ _____   ■ _____

■ _____   ■ _____

■ _____   ■ _____

■ _____   ■ _____

Psychological/emotional	Goals	Strategies

Psychological and emotional goals can include ensuring you do not allow poor self-esteem to make you abuse again at a specific date.

■ _____   ■ _____

■ _____   ■ _____

■ _____   ■ _____

■ _____   ■ _____

Cost-Benefit Pie Chart

Create a vivid picture of how substance usage is affecting your life.

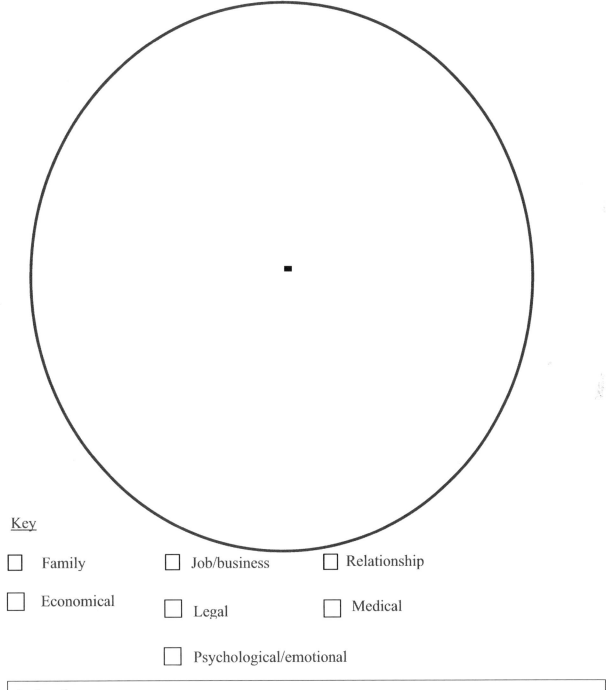

Key

☐ Family   ☐ Job/business   ☐ Relationship

☐ Economical   ☐ Legal   ☐ Medical

☐ Psychological/emotional

Instruction

What is the percentage of the effects of family, job/ business, relationship, finance, legal, medical, and emotional aspects of your life?

Create a pie chart with this circle by drawing lines from the center of the circle to the body of the circle.

Each section of the circle will represent the effects of substance abuse on these aspects of your life.

Do not forget to color the boxes in the key section below with the corresponding color.

Goals of Treatment

Set measurable goals with a time frame

Spiritual	Goals	Strategies

What spiritual goals do you have? You can decide to pray twice a day or keep a spiritual journal or any other thing that can help you in your progress.

Family	Goals	Strategies

You can decide to spend at least 2 hours daily engaging with your family or offer to be the one who picks up the kids from school.

My Daily Craving Record

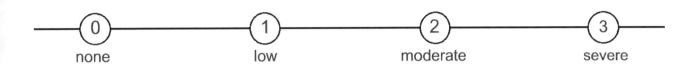

0	1	2	3
none	low	moderate	severe

Month _____

Day	Rating	Day	Rating	Day	Rating
1		11		21	
2		12		22	
3		13		23	
4		14		24	
5		15		25	
6		16		26	
7		17		27	
8		18		28	
9		19		29	
10		20		30/ 31	

Mental Health
Academy

Workbook

**Want to Learn More
About Mental Health
During a Pandermic
Like Covid-19?**

Scan QR to Download »

Week 1

Red Alerts to Relapse

Record your warning signs that can cause you to relapse

Physical

Emotional/psychological

Family/interpersonal relationship

Economic/job/business

Danger and Safe Zones

Describe in detail how your support group and risk group influence you. What role do they play in helping you to be drug-free or in increasing the risk of your substance abuse?

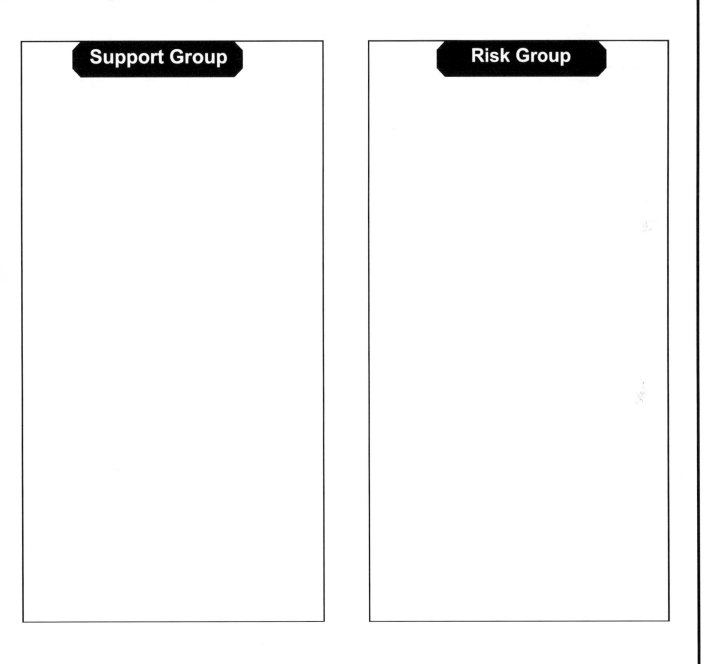

Support Group

Risk Group

Reviewing the Unsuccessful Attempts

(skip this sheet if this is your first attempt to be substance abuse free)

In the past, I tried several times to get rid of substance abuse.
Describe the unsuccessful attempts and failed coping strategies that
couldn't help

Review

Describe in detail what you have learned about yourself from previous sheets. What needs to be continued, what to be changed.

Dealing with High Risks

Describe in detail the top three high-risk and coping strategies that help you bring back to a safe zone.

High Risk 1

Coping Strategies

High Risk 2

Coping Strategies

High Risk 3

Coping Strategies

Automatic Thoughts and Behavior

At moderate to severe craving record your automatic thoughts and behavior

Trigger	Thought	Behavior
e.g. Spouse did pick the call	*e.g. he/she never picks my call not faithful enough, people are not trustworthy*	*e.g. I end up abusing*

Addiction Model

Activating Event
Trigger
argument with co-worker

Thought
I'm not good enough
I'm unable to maintain healthy
relationship

Emotion
feeling worthless, irritable, angry

Bodily Reaction
loss of apatite/ sleep

Behavior
negative behavior towards others
taking dose

Changing Thoughts

Activating Event
Trigger
argument with co-worker

Thought
I'm not good enough
I'm unable to maintain healthy relationship

Alternative Thought
everybody has the right to disagree, we should respect differences in opinions

Emotion
satisfied, relax

Bodily Reaction
normal

Behavior
positive towards others

My Thought Diary

Record your thoughts that are prone to relapse

Trigger _____

Thought	Emotion	Alternative Thought	Emotion

Trigger _____

Thought	Emotion	Alternative Thought	Emotion

Managing Emotions

Emotional instability is considered to be a high risk of substance abuse, mark the difficulty level of following emotions.

0	1	2	3
none	low	moderate	severe

Emotion	**Level of Difficulty**
	☐
Nervous	☐
Bored	☐
Happy/ excited	☐
Upset	☐
Angry	☐
Annoyed	☐
Tired	☐
Guilt	☐
Shame	☐
Depressed	☐
Feeling empty	☐

Managing Emotions

Enlist high-risk emotions and coping strategies

High Risk _____

Coping Strategies

High Risk _____

Coping Strategies

High Risk _____

Coping Strategies

Gratitude Week

I'm grateful for the little things in my life, e.g. I was able to reduce my wraps today

	Today I'm grateful for	**My BIG WIN today**
Day 1		
Day 2		
Day 3		
Day 4		
Day 5		
Day 6		
Day 7		

Review of Week 1

Enlist the coping strategies you have learned, the behaviors you have changed, positive activities you have acquired this week.

Week 2

Red Alerts to Relapse

Record your warning signs that can cause you to relapse

Physical

Emotional/psychological

Family/interpersonal relationship

Economic/job/business

Danger and Safe Zones

Describe in detail how your support group and risk group influence you. What role do they play in helping you to be drug-free or in increasing the risk of your substance abuse?

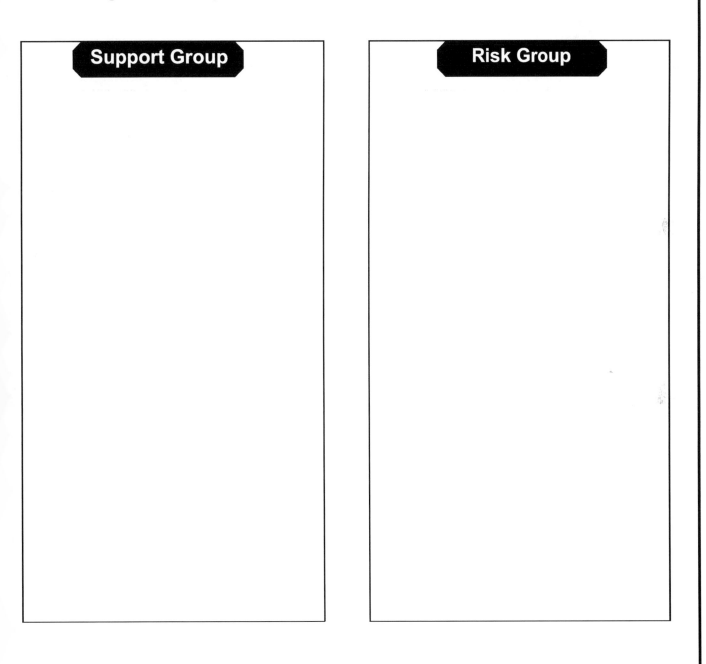

Support Group

Risk Group

Reviewing the Unsuccessful Attempts

(skip this sheet if this is your first attempt to be substance abuse free)

In the past, I tried several times to get rid of substance abuse.
Describe the unsuccessful attempts and failed coping strategies that couldn't help

Week 2 Review

Describe in detail what you have learned about yourself from previous sheets. What needs to be continued, what to be changed.

Dealing with High Risks

Describe in detail the top three high-risk and coping strategies that help you bring back to a safe zone.

High Risk 1

Coping Strategies

High Risk 2

Coping Strategies

High Risk 3

Coping Strategies

Automatic Thoughts and Behavior

At moderate to severe craving record your automatic thoughts and behavior

Trigger	Thought	Behavior
e.g. Spouse did pick the call	*e.g. he/she never picks my call not faithful enough, people are not trustworthy*	*e.g. I end up abusing*

Addiction Model

Activating Event
Trigger
argument with co-worker

Thought
I'm not good enough
I'm unable to maintain healthy
relationship

Emotion
feeling worthless, irritable, angry

Bodily Reaction
loss of apatite/ sleep

Behavior
negative behavior towards others
taking dose

Changing Thoughts

Activating Event
Trigger
argument with co-worker

Thought
I'm not good enough
I'm unable to maintain healthy relationship

Alternative Thought
everybody has the right to disagree, we should respect differences in opinions

Emotion
satisfied, relax

Bodily Reaction
normal

Behavior
positive towards others

My Thought Diary

Record your thoughts that are prone to relapse

Trigger _____

Thought	Emotion	Alternative Thought	Emotion

Trigger _____

Thought	Emotion	Alternative Thought	Emotion

Managing Emotions

Emotional instability is considered to be a high risk of substance abuse, mark the difficulty level of following emotions.

$$0 \quad 1 \quad 2 \quad 3$$

| none | low | moderate | severe |

Emotion	**Level of Difficulty**
	☐
Nervous	☐
Bored	☐
Happy/ excited	☐
Upset	☐
Angry	☐
Annoyed	☐
Tired	☐
Guilt	☐
Shame	☐
Depressed	☐
Feeling empty	☐

Managing Emotions

Enlist high-risk emotions and coping strategies

High Risk _____

Coping Strategies

High Risk _____

Coping Strategies

High Risk _____

Coping Strategies

Gratitude Week

I'm grateful for the little things in my life, e.g. I saw a beautiful bird on my balcony

	Today I'm grateful for	**My BIG WIN today**
Day 1		
Day 2		
Day 3		
Day 4		
Day 5		
Day 6		
Day 7		

Review of Week 2

Enlist the coping strategies you have learned, the behaviors you have changed, positive activities you have acquired this week.

Week 3

Red Alerts to Relapse

Record your warning signs that can cause you to relapse

Physical

Emotional/psychological

Family/interpersonal relationship

Economic/job/business

Danger and Safe Zones

Describe in detail how your support group and risk group influence you. What role do they play in helping you to be drug-free or in increasing the risk of your substance abuse?

Support Group	Risk Group

Reviewing the Unsuccessful Attempts

(skip this sheet if this is your first attempt to be substance abuse free)

In the past, I tried several times to get rid of substance abuse. Describe the unsuccessful attempts and failed coping strategies that couldn't help

Week 3 Review

Describe in detail what you have learned about yourself from previous sheets. What needs to be continued, what to be changed.

Dealing with High Risks

Describe in detail the top three high-risk and coping strategies that help you bring back to a safe zone.

High Risk 1 _____

Coping Strategies

High Risk 2 _____

Coping Strategies

High Risk 3 _____

Coping Strategies

Automatic Thoughts and Behavior

At moderate to severe craving record your automatic thoughts and behavior

Trigger	Thought	Behavior
e.g. Spouse did pick the call	*e.g. he/she never picks my call not faithful enough, people are not trustworthy*	*e.g. I end up abusing*

Addiction Model

Activating Event
Trigger
argument with co-worker

Thought
I'm not good enough
I'm unable to maintain healthy relationship

Emotion
feeling worthless, irritable, angry

Bodily Reaction
loss of apatite/ sleep

Behavior
negative behavior towards others
taking dose

Changing Thoughts

Activating Event
Trigger
argument with co-worker

Thought
I'm not good enough
I'm unable to maintain healthy relationship

Alternative Thought
everybody has the right to disagree, we should respect differences in opinions

Emotion
satisfied, relax

Bodily Reaction
normal

Behavior
positive towards others

My Thought Diary

Record your thoughts that are prone to relapse

Trigger _____

Thought	Emotion	Alternative Thought	Emotion

Trigger _____

Thought	Emotion	Alternative Thought	Emotion

Managing Emotions

Emotional instability is considered to be a high risk of substance abuse, mark the difficulty level of following emotions.

0	1	2	3
none	low	moderate	severe

Emotion   **Level of Difficulty**

Emotion	Level of Difficulty
Nervous	
Bored	
Happy/ excited	
Upset	
Angry	
Annoyed	
Tired	
Guilt	
Shame	
Depressed	
Feeling empty	

Managing Emotions

Enlist high-risk emotions and coping strategies

High Risk _____

Coping Strategies

High Risk _____

Coping Strategies

High Risk _____

Coping Strategies

Gratitude Week

I'm grateful for the little things in my life, e.g. I saw a beautiful bird on my balcony

	Today I'm grateful for	**My BIG WIN today**
Day 1		
Day 2		
Day 3		
Day 4		
Day 5		
Day 6		
Day 7		

Review of Week 3

Enlist the coping strategies you have learned, the behaviors you have changed, positive activities you have acquired this week.

Week 4

Red Alerts to Relapse

Record your warning signs that can cause you to relapse

Physical

Emotional/psychological

Family/interpersonal relationship

Economic/job/business

Danger and Safe Zones

Describe in detail how your support group and risk group influence you. What role do they play in helping you to be drug-free or in increasing the risk of your substance abuse?

Support Group

Risk Group

Reviewing the Unsuccessful Attempts

(skip this sheet if this is your first attempt to be substance abuse free)

In the past, I tried several times to get rid of substance abuse.
Describe the unsuccessful attempts and failed coping strategies that couldn't help

Week 4 Review

Describe in detail what you have learned about yourself from previous sheets. What needs to be continued, what to be changed.

Dealing with High Risks

Describe in detail the top three high-risk and coping strategies that help you bring back to a safe zone.

High Risk 1

Coping Strategies

High Risk 2

Coping Strategies

High Risk 3

Coping Strategies

Automatic Thoughts and Behavior

At moderate to severe craving record your automatic thoughts and behavior

Trigger	Thought	Behavior
e.g. Spouse did pick the call	e.g. he/she never picks my call not faithful enough, people are not trustworthy	e.g. I end up abusing

Addiction Model

Activating Event
Trigger
argument with co-worker

Thought
I'm not good enough
I'm unable to maintain healthy relationship

Emotion
feeling worthless, irritable, angry

Bodily Reaction
loss of apatite/ sleep

Behavior
negative behavior towards others
taking dose

Changing Thoughts

Activating Event
Trigger
argument with co-worker

Thought
I'm not good enough
I'm unable to maintain healthy relationship

Alternative Thought
everybody has the right to disagree, we should respect differences in opinions

Emotion
satisfied, relax

Bodily Reaction
normal

Behavior
positive towards others

My Thought Diary

Record your thoughts that are prone to relapse

Trigger _____

Thought	**Emotion**	**Alternative Thought**	**Emotion**

Trigger _____

Thought	**Emotion**	**Alternative Thought**	**Emotion**

Managing Emotions

Emotional instability is considered to be a high risk of substance abuse, mark the difficulty level of following emotions.

0	1	2	3
none	low	moderate	severe

Emotion | Level of Difficulty

Emotion	Level of Difficulty
	☐
Nervous	☐
Bored	☐
Happy/ excited	☐
Upset	☐
Angry	☐
Annoyed	☐
Tired	☐
Guilt	☐
Shame	☐
Depressed	☐
Feeling empty	☐

Managing Emotions

Enlist high-risk emotions and coping strategies

High Risk _____

Coping Strategies

High Risk _____

Coping Strategies

High Risk _____

Coping Strategies

Gratitude Week

I'm grateful for the little things in my life, e.g. I saw a beautiful bird on my balcony

	Today I'm grateful for	My BIG WIN today
Day 1		
Day 2		
Day 3		
Day 4		
Day 5		
Day 6		
Day 7		

Review of Week 4

Enlist the coping strategies you have learned, the behaviors you have changed, positive activities you have acquired this week.

Final Review

Enlist the coping strategies you have learned, the behaviors you have changed, positive activities you have acquired in general

Appendix
How to Use This Workbook

This self-help workbook contains worksheets that will help you in your fight against substance abuse. It can be used as an individual or as group therapy. It is a very simple workbook to use by anyone no matter their level of education and comprehension. We believe that substance abuse is not limited to any social class which is why we have made a lot of effort to keep it simple to use. However, to make it even easier for you, the explanations below will make it super easy to navigate your way around the workbook.

It starts with a section for doing a self-assessment or analysis to get to know more about yourself. This section contains a series of questions that you have to answer with a Yes or No answer. You are free to also include your questions if you feel that the questions are not enough for you or your group or doctor feels there are more relevant questions you need to answer.

The next section continues with the analysis of the problem. This section is subjective and needs you to be as honest as possible in stating how severe or bad you think the problem you are facing is. The severity is graded into low, moderate, high, severe, and extreme. And you will answer this question for health, psychological or emotions, job or business, relationship with others, economic, legal, and family.

What that means is that you will use that metric to measure your substance abuse has affected your health, psychological or emotions, job or business, relationship with others, economic, legal, and family.

Immediately following that is the motivation check. In this section, you have to state how interested you are in trying to stop this issue of substance abuse. So, prepare to state what your major reason is for wanting to fight this challenge. Are you doing it because someone else said so? Are you doing it just to get acceptance from someone or people? This section is very important because, without the right motivation, all of these will be a waste of time and money.

Following the motivation section is the section for analyzing the Cost and Benefit of following through with this program. The long-term and instant benefits are considered in this section. Every specific project must have a SMART goal. That means the goals must be Specific and not ambiguous, Measurable to determine if progress is being made. That is not all, the goal must also be Achievable and Realistic. This is not a time to state a goal that is not realistic considering other factors that may be at play. Not least important is that the goal must have a Time frame to achieve it.

Then we have a special pie chart for you to estimate by how much your substance abuse affects you and which of the different aspects is affected the most. The section provides you with the opportunity to create a visual image of the effect of substance abuse on you.

Then you get to record how strong your cravings for substance abuse are. Each of these has to be recorded daily. Even though the metric is listed as low, moderate, high, and severe, different people will have different ways of measuring what each of these terms means. Each person will have to define what qualifies as low, moderate, high, and severe. As you begin to progress, you will need to redefine these terms again because, we hope that after a while, what used to qualify as moderate can later be defined as severe because of how far you would have come in using the worksheets in this workbook.

With the personal profiling over, the worksheet will now begin at this point. To make you get the most out of this workbook, it has been divided into Week 1, Week 2, Week 3, and Week 4.

In each of those weeks, you will have to identify those things that increase your chances of relapsing despite all your efforts. These are like triggers, for example, certain kinds of friends, certain environments, certain moods, and emotions.

This will make way for you to document what your danger and safe zones are. The things that can and may help or support you in your plan to fight this substance abuse and those people or things that will make it difficult.

One thing you must know is that failure is bound to happen, very few people can succeed at the first attempt, so it is important to know why you failed so that you can pick yourself up and try again. We know this can happen, which is why we have provided a section for you to also document that. We want you to know that we are with you every step of the way and have anticipated some of the challenges you may face. So, do not be discouraged.

At the end of each week, we have 2 dedicated sections that allow you to leave a review of how well you were able to follow through with your plan for that week. In this workbook, you will also encounter one of the most important aspects of CBT therapy, which is the section that analyzes your thoughts and how they influence your emotions. You will find more details in the appendix of this book if you want more explanations.

You will also be introduced to the Addiction Model popularly used in CBT therapy. The Addiction Model is used in with the thought changing process to challenge the first thought that you had when you were triggered by your experience that made you crave substance abuse use.

In challenging your thoughts, you will start to create alternative thoughts to replace some of the initial thoughts that you unconsciously have each time you are triggered by an event. CBT believes that by controlling your thought process, you will become better at also controlling the kind of emotions you display when faced with a similar situation.

At the end of the process of redefining your thoughts and managing your emotions better, you will now have the opportunity to express your gratitude for the little steps you have undertaken and the baby progress you have made. Even though this section encourages you to tie your gratitude towards your fight against substance abuse addiction, you can however express gratitude on any aspect of your life. Thanksgiving is never too much.

Addiction Model Definitions

Activating Event Trigger

This important step is used to briefly describe the events that trigger you're your desire to abuse substance.

Example: At a social event today, everyone else was having a drink, I felt embarrassed and decided to also join.

Emotion

Emotion is what is used to describe what you feel activating event trigger you just experienced. Emotions are sometimes confused with thoughts which shouldn't be so. Emotions are the result of your what you have experienced.

Some words that you can use to explain your thoughts are available below:

Example:

- Jealous
- Joyful
- Cheerful
- Enraged
- Happy
- Annoyed
- Frightened
- Uneasy
- Unhappy
- Angry
- Nervous

- Euphoric
- Embarrassment
- Depressed
- Scared
- Mad
- Violation of personal rights
- Helpless
- Excited
- Tense
- Irritated
- Anxious
- Calm
- Frustrated
- Ashamed
- Discouraged
- Fear
- Insecurity
- Sad
- Panicky
- Flat
- Tired
- Exhilarate

Automatic Negative Thoughts

This next step is used to describe the first thoughts that entered your mind as a result of the trigger. It could well be a subconscious response of thoughts of something you have previously had.

Example: I feel like a miserable failure. People do not see anything good in me.

What Are Core Beliefs?

This important step is used to briefly describe the events that trigger you're your desire to abuse substance.

Core beliefs are assumptions and thoughts we have about ourselves, the people around us, and the world. These beliefs are usually deep-seated and often go unnoticed even though they tend to affect our lives constantly. It is mostly as a result of the belief that our thoughts and feelings affect us to such an extent that threatens to derail our success and happiness.

Common Core Beliefs That Can Hinder You

The belief that something is wrong with You

Core beliefs like this make you suffer from low self-esteem. It often prevents you from wanting to have any sort of friendship with people preferring instead to stay on your own, so that others do not notice what you perceive to be the things wrong with you. Beliefs like:

"I'm broken"

"Nothing about me is good, everything is wrong with me"

"I think I am no good"

"I think I am stupid and cannot make any right decision"

"I think I am worthless"

"Everyone around me has a better life than me"

"No one really knows I exist"

"I am such a bad person beyond redemption"

"I am a complete"

"Nothing I do ever goes right or works"

No One Can Love Me

Similar to the first one is the feeling of being unloved or unlovable. This can sometimes force you to avoid being in relationships so as to avoid experiencing your belief that you are not lovable or in some cases can make you try to force yourself on others even when they treat you badly or abuse you emotionally.

Thoughts associated with this belief include:

"I'm better off being on my own"

"I think I am boring"

"Everyone hates me"

"I can do things on my own"

"No one wants to understand me"

"Nobody wants me around them"

My Display of Love Seems Drive People Away from Me

Those with this kind of core belief often find themselves being scared of being rejected, prompting them to end relationships very early even when there is no need to do so.

This core belief is commonly associated with thoughts like:

"People end up abandoning me anyway"

"Loving someone is dangerous"

"When you love someone, you will get hurt"

"I have to be worthy to be loved"
"I can't find happiness if I am not with someone"
"People reject me"

We Live in a Dangerous World

This core belief is often associated with anxiety and fear so that your thoughts are only seen from a position of how to play safe based on your overexaggerated perception of danger. This will often prevent you from living up to your potential in life. Sometimes, it can lead you to be a control freak who wants to always be in control of everything without letting things go.
This belief will often result in thoughts like:
"No one is worthy of trust"
"Everyone is out to get me"
"I am not as powerful as others"
"I am helpless in most situations"
"I do not have the strength for anything"
"Being in control is the only way to survive"
"I have to always be on my guard"
"I should never leave myself vulnerable"
"I don't ever want to reveal who I really am"

I do not Consider Myself Good Enough

This type of core belief will usually make you either have low self-esteem which can lead to depression or make you feign perfectionist in an attempt to try to hide your low self-esteem and fears. In some other cases, you may have even given up trying to make yourself feel worthy and instead allow other people to manipulate and abuse you.

Core beliefs like this will manifest in situations like:

"I am incapable of changing"

"I am unskilled"

"I am a loser"

"I can never win no matter what I do"

"I am a born failure"

"There is really no need to make further efforts"

I'm Weird

This core belief tends to make you suffer from an extreme form of loneliness even when living in the midst of people. It will feel as if you do not even understand yourself. The manifestations of these core beliefs are noticeable in statements like:

"I do not know where I am from"

"I do not belong here"

"I feel like I come from a different planet"

"No one understands me"

"Something is not right with"

I Will Do Anything to Be Liked

This often stems from a core belief associated with childhood that only made a child feel loved only when they were good or acted in good behavior. This will make you not to be able to have steady relationships and identity issues. Some of these core beliefs associated with this core belief include:

"No one likes sad people"

"I cannot have bad thoughts"

"I am not loved when I am angry"

"When I do bad things, means I am a bad person"

I am Always at Fault

This core belief makes you not to have personal boundaries and an inability to say no to others. You will probably have relationships that are codependent. Common thoughts associated with this include:

"I do not want to hurt others"

"I am always wrong"

"I need to try harder"

"When I love people well enough, I will be able to fix them"

"I have to help everyone who comes my way"

"I have to be perfect"

I am a very Special Person

This type of core belief often results in great narcissism and grandiosity. This can result in you manipulating others and making others around you feel inferior and uneasy to be in your presence. It will often result in your not ever experiencing any form of true love and intimacy. Thoughts associated with this core belief include:

"I should be entitled to more"

"I deserve to have more attention"

"I shouldn't be criticized"

"I am superior to others"

"I am more intelligent than others"

Why Core Beliefs are Important

If sufficient time is not taken to try to dig out and have our negative core beliefs questioned, they will be capable of affecting the different decisions we make.

Analyzing Core Beliefs

Analyzing core beliefs will help us understand how they impact on our self-esteem, image, and future expectations. Negative core beliefs will distort our perception of the world and the way we see others around us. By taking this step, it now becomes possible to identify the core beliefs that have found a way to affect our thoughts, emotions, and behaviors.

How to Identify your Personal Core Beliefs?

In order to make the process easier for you, there are a few examples of questions you can ask to help you identify your views about yourself, others and the world around you.

Challenging your Core Beliefs

Many of the core beliefs we have, are neither true nor helpful, which is why a conscious effort has to be made to ensure that we challenge such beliefs and come up with ways to overcome them so that they do not overwhelm you. To evaluate and have your core belief challenged, you have to ask yourself a couple of questions. The essence of this exercise is to show that many of your unhelpful core beliefs are not only unhelpful but also not entirely true.

Questions to Challenge your Core Beliefs

What are my experiences that show that this belief isn't entirely true all the time?"
You use this exercise to list out as many of these experiences that you have. Make them as specific as possible in a factual way as if you were presenting it to a judge.
Do not forget to include even those experiences you are not sure are relevant to that scenario. When all the experiences have been listed, you can then proceed to develop an alternative and balanced core belief.
Next, you try and come up with what you consider to be more helpful and balanced core beliefs.

Made in the USA
Las Vegas, NV
19 April 2024

88899317R00050